Stop Battling Disease
&
Start Building Wellness

Stop Battling Disease
&
Start Building Wellness

Your Guide to Extraordinary Pet Care

Tonijean Kulpinski, CBHC, BCHP, AADP,
Board-Certified Holistic Drugless Practitioner

Special Addition
The Most Beautiful Love Story

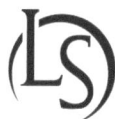

LEON SMITH
PUBLISHING

Images by Vladimir Kulpinski

ISBN: 978-1-945446-79-5

First, this book is dedicated to my beloved golden retriever and handsome prince, Peanut, who went to be with the Lord August 9, 2019, at 3:03 in the afternoon. This truly was the saddest and most painful day of my life. Peanut, you were my best friend, my soul mate, and my twenty-four-hour buddy. I love you more than words can express, and I thank you for the beautiful years that you've given me. I can only hope that I have blessed you half as much as you have blessed me. You truly live on in my heart each and every day. Knowing that I have eternity to look forward to when we reunite over the rainbow bridge, gives me such peace.

My dear husband, my human soul mate, my best friend, my lover, and my partner in life. I cannot describe in words what you mean to me. We've been through it all and yet God found a way to keep us strong and together. I look forward to eternity with you, loving you forever.

My precious Michaela. I am so proud of the beautiful young woman you've become. You are more than everything I could ever hope for in a daughter. You have grown so beautifully into all that God has created you to be. My life is complete with you by my side, my baby girl, my best friend. Thank you for making Mama so proud. I love you all the way to the moon and back.

Michael Dubois, you are most definitely part of our family. Peanut loved you so much, especially because he knew exactly how much you loved him. Our Milky Way has grown very fond of you and you of him. I could not have asked God for a better man for my daughter. Thank you for loving and respecting her exactly the way you do. I love you like a son.

I thank you, my heavenly Father God for continuing to bless me with both knowledge and wisdom on my holistic journey, helping others heal themselves, including our furry loved ones.

To All the Pets We've Loved Before Who Have Crossed Over The Rainbow Bridge

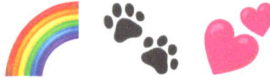

Peanut, Finn, Bummer, Tuffy, Otis, Lady, Ginger, Princess, Benjamin, Lilly, Teddy, Lilly, Petey, Boobe, Skippy, Dot, Max, and Bella.

To All the Pets We Love Who Are Still Here
Milky Way, Chase, Wesley, Lilly, Bailey, Yankee

Contents

Praise for *Stop Battling Disease & Start Building Wellness*

"This is the long-awaited third book in the series, *Stop Battling Disease & Start Building Wellness*. In this *Guide to Extraordinary Pet Care*, you will learn what you should feed your pets, supplements that should be given, and much, much more.

People comment all the time about my dog, Bailey and how healthy and his shiny coat is and that he is full of boundless energy. This is due to following the protocols in Toni's book.

Toni, thank you for sharing your knowledge with the world! My family and of course Bailey are 'fur-ever' grateful!"

— Nicole Roberts
Special Education Teacher
and....
Believer in all things are possible

"I first met Tonijean during my long journey to heal my daughter, Isabel, who suffered with eczema for the first twelve years of her life. Thanks to Tonijean, who answered my prayers, Isabel is completely healed from within. This is a gift I will forever cherish. During our many visits to Tonijean's house, Isabel and I saw firsthand her deep love for Peanut and now, Milky Way. I have worked in the veterinary field for over twenty years. Every day I witness dogs and cats suffering from diseases like arthritis, allergies, cancer, and auto-immune disease. Tonijean's book, *Stop Battling Disease & Start Building Wellness: Your Guide to Extraordinary Pet Care*, will allow you to transform the health of your pet so that you can love and enjoy them for as long as possible free of disease."

— Dr. Christine Barnhorst, DVM, Owner of Walker Valley Veterinary Hospital Nutrition & Wellness Center

"Good nutrition is the key to a healthy and long life for our fur-babies. I support animal rights and holistic health, and I am thrilled that Tonijean chose to share her journey with Peanut and honor him by revealing so many easy to follow, wholesome recipes for animals. Her guidance and passion for God's world translates into each ingredient and page of her book. As an animal trainer and behaviorist, I have witnessed firsthand how these foods can lift a dog's life up with good health and increase positive behaviors. We all want our pups to have the best, and knowledge is power. This book gives you that power.

— Larell Green, CPDI, CPTI, AT,
Accredited Dog Behaviorist and Educator

"I am excited to add Tonijean's latest book, *Stop Battling Disease & Start Building Wellness: Your Guide to Extraordinary Pet Care* to my collection. I keep these books prominently displayed on my bookshelf as I view them as my very own personalized holistic physician's desk reference. They are always my first reach for any questions that arrive. I am lucky enough to call Tonijean my dear friend as well and having that access to her rolodex-like knowledge is a blessing from heaven. Tonijean seems to have an unending need to make our world a better place. She clearly has a calling. God chose her to bless us and now our beloved pets!"

— Felicia M Dopico, Author of *Journey Out of Egypt*

Acknowledgments

Mom, I first want to thank you for being the most selfless, loving mother I could ever hope for. Thank you for loving me unconditionally. You are the solid rock of our family and the glue that holds us all together. I love you, my mommy, today and forever.

My amazing sister Francesca, We did it—two bestselling authors— yay! Fran, you are my best friend, my sister, my soul sister, my world. I'm so very proud of you for so many reasons and I could never imagine my life without you. Thank you for your unconditional love and always being there no matter what. I love you with every beat of my heart.

My dear brother Richard, I'll say it again, you have believed in me right from the start of this incredible journey, I thank you with all my heart for the countless hours you've dedicated teaching me exactly what I needed to learn and supporting all my goals. I love you beyond words.

My precious niece Michelle, you are such a gift from God. You are not only my niece, but my dear friend. I thank you for your words of wisdom and encouragement to continue this journey. I love you more than you can ever imagine.

Christian, Selah, and Elion, you three are the best little—getting bigger—nieces and nephews that I could ever ask God for. I love you all so very much. Please know to follow your hearts' desires and make all your dreams come true. Look to God first in everything.

Franca Amato Sanchez, thank you, my precious sister, for believing in me, and for the countless hours sharing each other's dreams. I love you, doll.

My incredible, amazing, beautiful friend Nicole Roberts, I don't even know where to begin because there's so much that you've done for me. I am forever grateful, blessed, and honored to call you my friend. I love you as if you were my other sister. Thank you for your continued friendship and for every wonderful moment. I love you beyond words.

Christine Felicello, you are truly my family. We have been through so much together—the good, the scary, the happy, and the sad, and I wouldn't change one moment of it. I love you so much and I thank you for your twenty-four-hour love and support. Christine, you have been there for me through everything, and I don't know how I'd ever live this life without you. With much love and gratitude for a lifetime of friendship with you, my sister.

Dana Swensen, you are without a doubt my family. I love you sooo much; you are an angel to me right here on this earth. You have grown so much over the years into all that God has created you to be. Looking at a longggg friendship in our own world. LOL

Donna Pizza, we go back quite some time and I've so enjoyed the beautiful ride. *Family* is what comes to mind when I think of you. I am so proud of all that you've become through this beautiful journey called life. With much love.

My dear friend Connie Grimaldi, I have so many awesome memories with you, especially Halloween. LOL. You are extremely special and very important to me, like no other. I LOVE you and look forward to all our fun and even sad times together because we know exactly how to comfort one another.

Kathy Meroney, *angel* is still my very first thought when I think of you. You have every characteristic of a true-life angel. You, Fran, and I go way back; our journeys reflect into my thoughts like a movie. We've had great times and difficult times, but because of our strong, godly friendship we not only got through them, we got the victory. I love you more than you can even imagine, no different from a family member.

Lennis Giansante Lubrano, to this day, I still can't thank you enough for all your continued prayers, for believing in me and foreseeing the vision of what God had in store for my future. I thank God I listened to you. I love you so much, my beautiful dear Lennis.

Lisa Buldo, I am so grateful for Trinity Broadcast Network; without them, I'd never have met you. Thank you for your friendship, prayers, love, and support and for always having me on your incredible broadcast. You have blessed me tremendously. I love you Lisa.

Felicia and Abigail Dopico, thank you for your continued love and support and for the incredible friendship we have built. Your love for the Lord shines through you and in all that you do. I am forever blessed to call you my friends. With much love.

Caroline Krieger and Jeff Petkevicius, I don't even know where to begin. You both have touched my heart so deeply, and I've grown to love you both like family. I love how you love the Lord in all that you do. I look forward to a lifetime of great friendships and success on the path God has set us out to do. With much love.

Patty Bishop, you mean more to me than I think you even realize. Please know how much I absolutely adore you. Thank you for your love for the Lord and all your wisdom that you so generously share. With much love.

Michelle Chirigliano, I can't begin to thank you enough for all your love and support during my grieving of my beloved Peanut. I also want to thank you for your beautiful, loving friendship.

Jody Carson, thank you so much for your kindness and friendship. I will always carry a special place in my heart for you, for being there during my most intense time of grief. With much love.

Kristin Craig, you were there for me when my beloved Peanut passed, and I am ever so grateful to you. You have shown and given me so much friendship and love throughout the time you've been my client. I have grown to love you.

Nancy Pierro, I thank you so much for all your love and support, for always attending my events, sending me clients, and believing in me. Love you, my dear friend.

Keith and Maura Leon, first and foremost, I thank you for everything that you've taught me on this incredible journey. You are two of the kindest and most selfless people I know. I've truly grown to love you both. I am forever changed due to our journey together from the very beginning until now. Love and many blessings to you always.

As for everyone else at Babypie Publishing: Karen Burton, Autumn Carlton, and Heather Taylor, thank you for all your hard work with editing and all the additional phases that have brought my work from manuscripts to incredible bestselling books. Much love, tremendous gratitude, and many blessings to each of you.

Charice Damiani, I thank you again for your outstanding friendship. I am ever so blessed to have you in my life. With much love.

My beautiful and dear friend, Laura Thompson, you are most definitely my soul sister. We go back quite some time, and it just keeps on getting better. From one author to another, I'll love and cherish you forever. With much love.

Angela Locker, you and I could probably write a book together, and I'm sure it would be a bestseller. LOL. I can't thank you enough for believing in me, for your support, love, and amazing friendship. I love you my beautiful friend (Dog).

Tammi Boyd, I am so blessed to call you my friend. Thank you for all your continued love and support. I pray an abundance of blessings upon you and your family. Love you.

Cameron Cushing, I owe you another huge thank you, not only for your beautiful friendship, but for leading me to Babypie Publishing. I am so grateful and blessed with your friendship. Much love and abundant blessings to you, my dear friend.

Lisa Love, I am so grateful to have been blessed with your friendship. You are such a shining light in a dark world. You're beautiful in and out and I hope that one day you decide to put all your impeccable talent into a book. With much love.

Larell Green, I am so happy that I walked into PetSmart a few years ago because I met an amazing new person whom I now call a friend. I adore you, girlfriend, and I cannot ever repay you for all that you've done for me. With MUCH love.

Regina Cieslak, You are one amazing person and I am blessed to have you in my life. I pray a multitude of continued blessings upon you. Love you, my dear friend.

Debby Wimberly, my walking partner, my wonderful friend, the piece that makes my circle complete. I am forever grateful. I very much look forward to a lifetime of friendship with you my beautiful and amazing friend. With much love.

Everyone else, I thank you all for choosing my books for yourself and for your human and furry family of loved ones. May God bless you with extraordinary health all the days of your lives.

Prologue: A Letter to Peanut

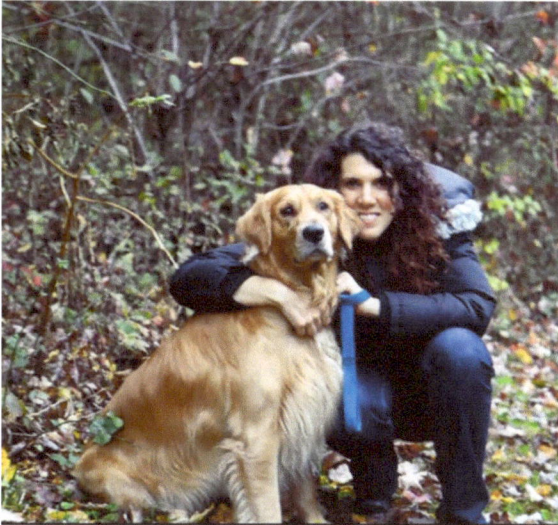

Mama and Peanut

Until one has loved an animal, a part of one's soul remains unawakened.
~ Anatole France. ☺

I don't even know where to begin. One full year without you here has been one of the most painful experiences I've ever endured. Peanut, you were my twenty-four-hour buddy, my soul's best friend. We were the perfect fit. You were there for me when no one else was, and when others were there, so were you. You were always there! So how do I go on from here? Losing you is certainly not something I will get over or even get through; I just keep going. The pain of grief doesn't end; it continues to grow the longer you're not here.

My beloved boy, I thank you for choosing our family as your family and blessing us with the most wonderful, selfless, incredible, joyous, amazing, happiest, funniest, silliest, most loving years of our lives. I will remember you with a smile; you shaped my heart into love.

I know you know how much Mama loves you. I kissed you a thousand times a day. My beautiful boy, Mama dedicated this book to you so the world can see true love through our eyes.

Eternity is forever; there is no end. Knowing you are waiting there for me and our family to return to each other one day gives me the peace and comfort I need to move forward.

Loving an animal awakens one's soul to a higher love, a love beyond human understanding, and you, my boy, enabled me to do just that.

I'll love you today and fur-ever ❤🐾❤

Peanut, you were such a blessing in my life; how fortunate I am to have been blessed with you. You gave all of us unconditional love each and every day—constant joy, happiness, loyalty, comfort, laughter, and warmth. What a wonderful and beautiful life we shared, especially trips to Hawthorne Valley Farm where I think you believed you owned the place. You loved to run freely on the beautiful, green, plush acres and swim in the lakes and ponds.

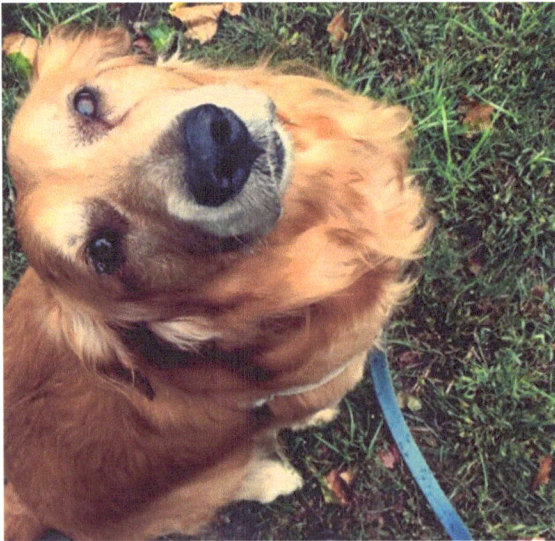

Peanut at Farm

Just before we would go to *your* farm, I would always say, "Do you wanna go bye-bye in the car and show Daddy how you swim?" You would go crazy and run all around the house and then wait by the door. Our countless memories of you bring such joy to our hearts.

One of the most difficult things I've ever gone through was losing you, my beloved boy. The pain doesn't ever go away; it deepens with each passing day that you're not physically here. With your passing, Peanut, I lost a large part of me, which shows as a huge hole in my heart. But then you sent me Milky Way, the English cream golden retriever we welcomed on September 5, 2019, at eleven weeks old, who has already started to fill that hole.

Once someone has had the good fortune to share a true love affair with a golden retriever, one's life and one's outlook is never quite the same.
~ Betty White

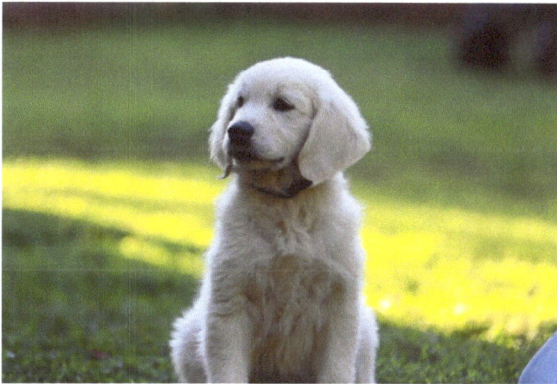

Puppy Milky Way

Peanut, you will *never* be replaced, but in honor of you, I carry our love to the beautiful precious Milky Way, and I look forward to building many memories with him. As I get to know Milky Way, it is so evident that your spirit is shining through him.

You think dogs will not be in heaven? I tell you,
they will be there long before any of us.
~ Robert Louis Stevenson

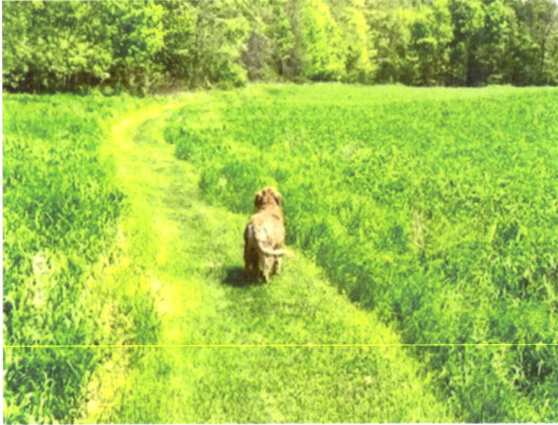

Peanut Running Free

Introduction

Welcome back! I'd like to congratulate you for completing my first and second books, *STOP Battling Disease & Start Building Wellness: Your Guide to Extraordinary Health and STOP Battling Disease & Start Building Wellness: Your Guide to Extraordinary Meals, The Cookbook,* in my *Stop Battling Disease* series. If you have not yet read either book, please visit Amazon or Tonijeanapproved.com where you can order your copies and enjoy the entire series.

Although I have such compassion for the human race and do all I do to see the world a healthier and happier place, my focus includes all non-human creatures as well.

I am a total animal lover and would absolutely risk my own life to save a vulnerable animal. I wrote this book not only because of my love and respect for our furry loved ones, but because there is so much misinformation out there on how to feed and care for your pet. As a practitioner, I have also had the honor of successfully working with countless animal patients, reversing some detrimental health issues that were the result of incorrect veterinary advice.

Animals are uniquely created by our loving God, and I wholeheartedly believe they are put here to teach us how to love more deeply, how to be more patient, and how to connect with and respect the Earth and all living things. Animals love unconditionally and deserve that exact kind of love in return. This love includes how we feed and nurture them, because a healthy pet is a happy pet.

Chapter One

The Most Beautiful Love Story

If you've ever been privileged to own and love a cat or a dog,
then you know real, unconditional love.

Please allow me to share with you . . . "The Most Beautiful Love Story"

Have you ever heard anyone say the words: *It's just a dog?*

Words cannot describe the pain my family and I have endured over the physical loss of our best friend, soulmate, companion, family member, fur-baby, and fur-son.

The relationship that I personally had with my boy Peanut goes far beyond what words can even express. He came into my life after I had completely healed myself holistically from cancer, had lost an organ, and was battling other extreme health issues.

Saying Peanut rescued me is an understatement. Peanut restored me, renewed me, and rejuvenated me. He taught me and my family how to love even deeper than we ever knew possible. Peanut touched the lives of countless people exactly where they needed his touch. Imagine *just a dog* teaching us how to be human. Well, Peanut did exactly that.

He also gave me the courage to bless this message of health and self-love that I experience each and every day to multitudes of people that desperately need it. Peanut has not only healed me on so many levels, but his teaching of love and communication exalted my personal relationship with my husband.

Reflecting on every single day with Peanut was nothing short of intense joy, optimal mental and physical health, extraordinary happiness, and constant smiles: the car rides, swimming, ball playing, stick throwing, presents, treats, and tons of nature adventures. The memories of quiet time of hugging and cuddling are memories of the most pure love one could ever imagine.

Oh, how blessed we all were!

Every single day with my boy, whether I was having a bad day or a good day, was always a great day because of Peanut's constant expression of unconditional love. There wasn't one single day that I didn't kiss my boy and tell him how much I loved him. We had a beautiful life together. I like to call our life together . . . "The Most Beautiful Love Story"

Our love was the kind where you love and don't want anything in return but love. Just the way love should be. I took optimal care of my boy because I'd have it no other way. *It's what you do.* I respected his body by giving him a tremendous amount of love, belly rubs, doggie massages, and the best source of homemade food and supplements.

I have found tremendous peace and strength through this journey. I know my boy is here with me, just in a different form. I feel him everywhere, and the signs he's giving me are nothing short of angelic miracles. He and I will reunite one day, and what a beautiful reunion it will be. I am finally in a beautiful place of peace because the life we had and shared was beyond magical, and I will reflect only on that.

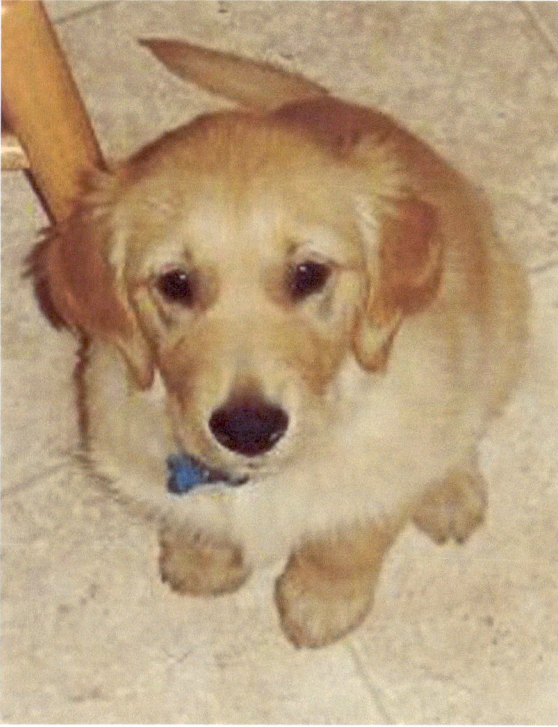

Peanut Puppy

HOW IT ALL BEGAN

Peanut, our beautiful golden retriever, came into our lives at the age of merely eight weeks old. My daughter and I wanted a golden badly, so I had secretly searched for a private breeder that was not a puppy mill. I found this wonderful lady named Mary in Unadilla, NY. I had never heard of this town, but it was just outside Oneonta, so that was familiar.

My daughter, Michaela, already had the name Peanut picked out, just in case we found a golden. Michaela knows that I will travel far to get real food, so I told her we were going on a trip to pick up fresh ground jungle peanut butter. We arrived at our destination three hours later, and we got the biggest and fluffiest golden—by her request—in a litter of ten. There he was, Peanut, waiting for his fur-ever home with the Kulpinski family. The rest is now history and lives in our hearts fur-ever.

My best friend, Peanut, is the dog that came into my life and rescued me. His love enabled me to be all that I am today. Peanut fit right in with our family; we all, including my husband, instantly fell in love.

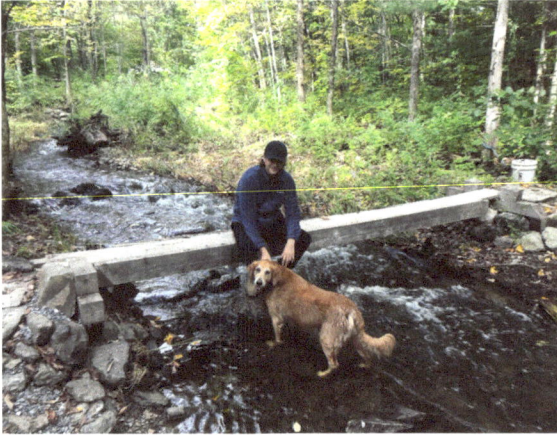

Peanut and Vladimir

LOVE, GRIEF, AND PEACE

This pain is not the absence of peace; it's merely a symptom of grieving your physical loss, but peace knowing your spirit is right here.

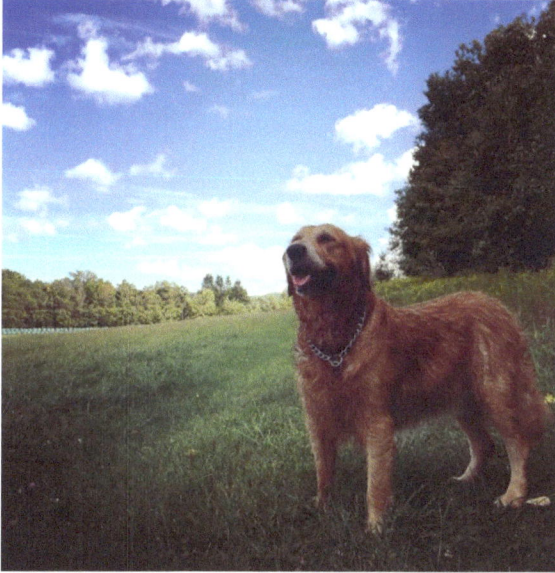

Peanut's Spirit

The pain of losing our precious Peanut has been extremely overwhelming, but we are blessed to have so many incredibly beautiful people in our lives who touched us in such tremendous ways.

The day that our boy passed, I felt that I couldn't go on and continue on the healing path where God has placed me. I felt I could never get through this pain and lead people in health the way I do. I was about to give up. Through all the beautiful prayers, heartfelt messages, and sympathy cards, I snapped out of that depression almost instantly.

That's the power of God!

Each person has made me realize that Peanut, my best friend and inspiration all these years, is still with me and continues to be my inspiration. I feel his spirit all around me strongly, and what a wonderful feeling of peace and joy it brings me.

Of course, the enemy would try to break me so I would no longer be able to continue to lead the masses to health freedom, but God has a different plan. *Nothing* will stop me from my passion and life's purpose, from continuing my journey to restore the mental and physical health of this nation and world, one life at a time.

Peanut has been the vessel that God placed in my life to rescue me so I could be all that God has called me to be. I will live on through his legacy of true love.

I have not had one bad memory with my boy. He was always healthy almost until his last breath. He ran and played every single day of his life. No hip dysplasia, no cataracts, no arthritis, no joint issues, no skin issues ever—not even one cold or ear infection in his entire life. Every single day of Peanut's life, I told him how much I loved him, and he would look at me with such admiration. There honestly wasn't one day that I didn't kiss him and say, "I love you so much." Sometimes, he'd sigh as if he was saying: *Oh no, not again!*

Peanut was happy and joyful each and every day of his life, and he touched the lives of countless people. As I went back to seeing patients after his passing, there wasn't one person who didn't shed tears for our boy. They all claimed that Peanut was a huge part of their healing. I will carry on in the memory of Peanut and rise up even higher as the holistic practitioner, leader, and healer that I am set out to be.

I thank God each and every day that he chose Peanut for me and my family and chose us for Peanut. I would not be who or where I am today without everything that Peanut has taught me.

Thank you, Peanut, for all your love, all your love, all your love.

A dog is the only thing on Earth that loves you more than he loves himself.
~ Josh Billings

HE SUPPLIES ALL OUR NEEDS.

I would like to share with you how magnificent God truly is. In God's pharmacy, there's a remedy for everything!

I suffered intense pain from the loss of my beloved Peanut to the point where I was saying that the only way I can describe my pain was that it was as if my heart were bleeding. I was desperate to find some relief from this deep pain but certainly didn't want to take some harsh prescription. I then researched in hopes to find an effective remedy from nature.

I discovered a product by Siddha, called *Cell Salts and Flower Essences: Grief and Loss*. I began taking it as directed and although my thoughts were sad, it helped tremendously. A feeling of peace came over me, along with all the outpouring of love and prayers from many. As time went by and I had moments of deep sadness, I would take the product again to receive the same calming and peaceful results.

When I looked at the ingredients in this product, I discovered the main ingredient is an herb called *bleeding heart*. ♥ Wow, how amazing is our God!

Thank you, Father God, for always giving us all that we need, exactly when we need it.

LOVE AND SUPPORT

Here are just a few of the many messages we received from great and very dear friends. We found comfort in them, and you might too.

You need to know that others care . . . but words seem so shallow at a time like this. Peanut became a friend to all of us through you and the sharing of his pictures, videos, his toys. We all loved him. He was a very special boy and became an internet celebrity! I know today you are crushed, and the pain is so real and so deep that you don't know how to carry on. In time, others will grow weary hearing about it or seeing your tears. But that's okay, you take all the time you need to cry and to grieve. BUT, you keep in mind that this is a temporary place; you are not allowed to dwell there! There is great danger in staying in places that attract the spirit of depression and others to join. Jesus must be your focus and strength. I have such great compassion for you and empathy as well, but I love you enough to say that you are called, and you have many depending on you. You must not allow this to consume you or it will. You are so loved and cared about. I know there must be multitudes praying for you right now and your family. Your precious baby loved you and desired to please you, and you loved him beyond measure— that was evident. Allow yourself to weep and to love and to come to grips with reality once again. My precious friend, remember when we are weak, He is made strong. Lean hard into Jesus and your friends that know Him and love you! Continual prayers and hugs! ♥

~ Patty 'n Ronnie Bishop

Peanut
Your fur baby went beyond companion,
His overwhelming love for you could fill a canyon,
You feel so empty; your heart completely broken,
As you look for your Peanut and his name softly spoken,
His scent alive and still present all around you,
As you hold his favorite toy that you knew he loved to chew.
You hear him running through the house,
As you place your hand upon your blouse,
You hear sounds, the jingling of his collar, his familiar bark,
As you close your eyes and remember him playing in the park,
He knew you, every step, every look, every emotion,
Communication with words never spoken, silence in motion.
All this love for you, Peanut carried within,
Came from the Heaven above, where Peanut had been,
Peanut chose you for a reason,
He spent his life loving you through every season,

He left because he knew you were ready,
His job complete, you, no longer unsteady,
A vessel he was, to teach and learn,
To receive nothing in return.
His one greatest gift was how to give love,
To show love, to share love, which he had a lot of,
He was on a mission from above,
So simple, unconditional, precious love,
He knew when you were sad and unhappy,
But rejoiced with you when you were sassy and laughing.
We often realize later on, what an impact was left behind,
Peanut will never be gone really; his love exists within, just look for the
signs.
You may not feel it now, but know that he has made you stronger,
His purpose, whatever it may had been, needed no longer.
I believe God puts angels in our lives,
No matter the size, shape or form, to somehow help us thrive,
I look at you, Toni, and I see glorious light, love as God's clinician,
Our Lord chose you for true discipleship in your mission.
Peanut was a part of God's goal for you,
Do grieve, mourn, miss your Peanut and get through to continue your
work giving others hope,
For healing, for releasing our fears and to cope.
We all love you for who you are and your kindness and gentle touch,
For you inspire and are needed so very much,
So full of gratitude for your knowledge and wisdom,
As you continue God's work and fulfill your vision.
When you feel yourself slipping, do not fear,
Your angels are watching and Peanut is surely near,
So, with a pat on his head and a whisper and a kiss,
Your sweet Peanut will surely be missed.

~ written with much love and empathy
by Michelle A. Cirigliano

HEALING

I am ready for God to raise me up to the highest level, not have the enemy take me down!

I am still in some level of pain every day, and that is an emotion I know will never go away—that's okay. Peanut and I had an unconditional, beautiful love that will never fade, and what gives me peace is what I want to bless forward to you.

The loss of our furry family members is a time of sadness we all go through as animal lovers/owners. The pain is unbearable. Every day, I see people who either have just lost their furry friend or are going through the end stage of their pet's life. If you are in this position, please know this: these loved ones were meant to be with you and you with them. There are no coincidences, only GOD-incidences. During these sad days, you must reflect on the wonderful and amazing life that you so graciously gave your friends, as well as all the beautiful gifts they have given you.

The quality of life in their short time here on Earth is greater than the length. They are not supposed to be here that long because, in reality, they are angels who teach us how to love more deeply and to fulfill our spiritual needs—to teach, heal, and rescue us on so many different levels. Oh, how I know this to be true.

My Words to You in Your Loss

I feel my Peanut near me every day and that brings me joy and a smile. I know that he has just paved the way for me and our other loved ones to use when it's our time to join him in eternity.

Look at your fur-baby's passing as a blessing; see that not only were they ready but they knew you were complete in all that you should be.

Remember all the laughter they gave, the hugs and kisses that you surely carry on in your heart fur-ever.

Your furry loved ones are certainly not gone; they live right here in your heart. They are running free, happy, and healthy, waiting for you to one day rekindle your love in eternity, FUR-EVER.

Remember, eternity has no end. That's the most beautiful gift that God has blessed us all with.

Please bless your love forward and love another furry friend. I know that's exactly what they want you and me to do. When Milky Way sees me crying, he runs over to comfort me. It's the best feeling. I've grown to love him so much, yet somehow, I also loved him even before he got here.

Even in the midst of my deepest pain, I'm sending my love and many hugs to all that have gone through this, past or present. My heart weeps with yours.

I hear you in the wind. I feel you in my heart. I see your reflection in my tears.

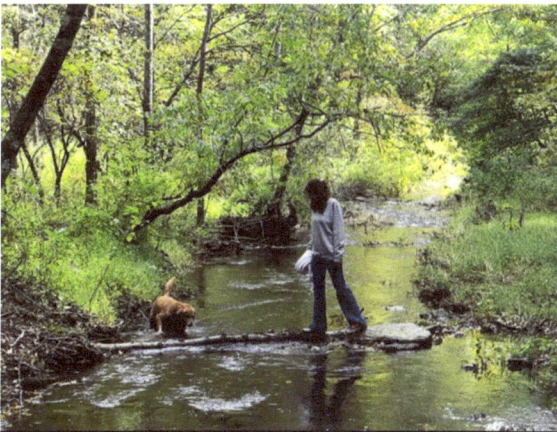

I Hear You in the Wind

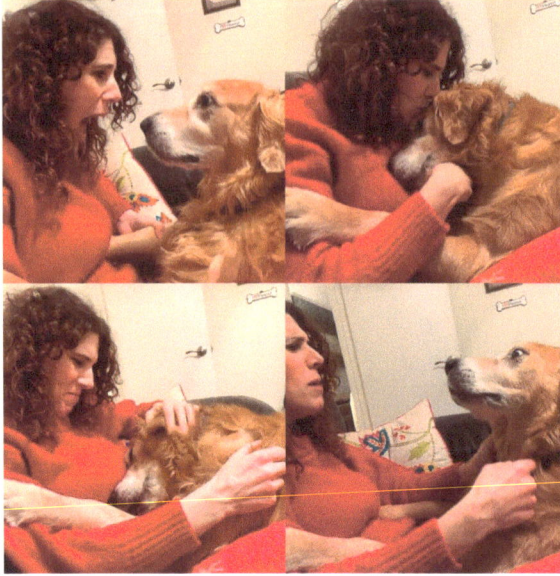

I love you every day

Peanut, I love you every day of my life and look forward to the day we run toward each other when I come home to our final happy place over the rainbow.

In His hand is the life of every living thing and the breath of all mankind.
Job 12:10 (ESV)

Your righteousness is like the highest mountains,
your justice like the great deep.
You, Lord, preserve both people and animals.
Psalm 36:6 (NIV)

TO PEANUT FROM MILKY WAY

My dear, beloved brother Peanut, I see our mama tear up every day as she talks to me about you. I also see the most intense depth of love for you in her eyes. It's during these exact moments when I need to keep Mama laughing, as she chases me all around the house trying to get a shoe, sock, or dishtowel from my mouth. LOL

I want you to know that I'm taking great care of all of them as they are taking such great care of me. I can see how much our entire family loves you.

Thank you for lending me your toys and bowls. I even use your leash from time to time although, out of Mama's love for me, she bought me my very own stuff too.

I have a wonderful life here living in your legacy, and somehow we all just know that you're right here together with us, as we will always be one loving family.

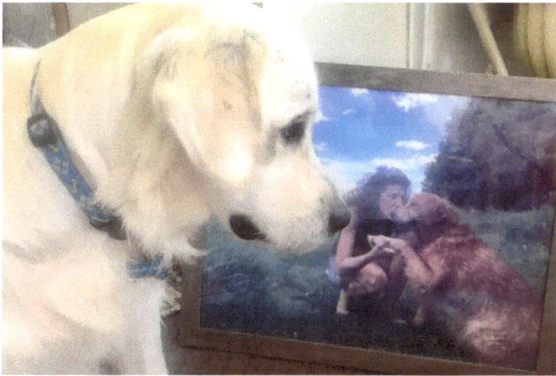

Letter to Peanut from Milky Way

Chapter Two

What Your Dog and Cat Should Eat

A hundred years from now, it will not matter the sort of house I lived in, what my bank account was, or the car I drove . . . but the world may be different because I was important in the life of the animals and the creatures on this Earth.

~ Author Unknown

Our furry friends give us love and devotion unconditionally all their lives. One of the ways we can show our love for them is by supplying them with the right foods. Remember, a healthy pet is a happy pet!

Like humans, our furry loved ones also suffer from health problems from time to time. We currently see a rise in many pet health conditions, including:

- Cancer
- Digestive issues
- Abnormal growths
- Thyroid problems
- Bad breath
- Teeth and gum issues
- Hot spots (red, itchy areas of skin)
- Fur loss
- Skin allergies
- Ear infections
- Diabetes

I believe wholeheartedly that diet plays a huge role in the rise of these conditions and a role in some forms of bad behavior.

Consequently, if you're feeding your animal genetically engineered or pesticide-laden foods, these sources may very well be the hidden culprit in your pet's health issues. As a naturopathic practitioner, I treat many people with a variety of health conditions. In addition to my human patients, I have also had the opportunity to successfully help dogs and cats regain their God-given health.

Unfortunately, it is my professional opinion that many licensed veterinarians are giving incorrect health advice, which has not only hindered healing but has prolonged health problems. Many of these problems can be healed naturally. I do understand the importance of emergency pet care in the event of a serious issue. It breaks my heart to know how many dogs and cats go into their veterinarian's office for various health conditions and receive harsh drugs, including steroids, which inhibit the body's ability to heal. In addition, pet foods suggested by veterinarians often contain a host of synthetic vitamins, chemical fertilizers, and other harmful ingredients.

On a better note, I am blessed and grateful to be able to deliver the true message of health so your furry baby can heal successfully and enjoy great health. You're probably wondering: *What is the best pet food on the market?* Well, although I will give my top suggestions, I believe there really isn't a perfect pet food; therefore, I suggest making your own. Let's first talk about what we should *not* be feeding our dogs and cats.

Here is a list of foods that are healthy for humans, but are potentially harmful for our four-legged family members due to a photochemical that may compromise their immune system.

HARMFUL FOODS

- Macadamia nuts
- Some varieties of avocado, such as those grown in the West Indies and the larger avocado varieties found in the state of Florida. Haas avocados are perfectly fine.
- Grapes and raisins
- Chocolate, including cacao

Most of you will probably be shocked to learn about some foods that are actually healthy for your pet, since you may have been told otherwise.

HEALTHY FOODS FOR FURRY LOVED ONES

- Fruit—yes, you heard that right
- Vegetables
- All types of potatoes: red skin, sweet, heirloom, yellow skin
- Lentils
- Quinoa
- Rolled oats
- Brown and wild rice
- Buckwheat
- Barley
- Millet
- Grass-fed beef
- Grass-fed lamb
- Pastured chicken
- Wild fish, with scales and fins
- Pastured eggs

- Almond butter, cashew butter, walnut butter, and jungle peanut butter
- Unrefined oils, such as coconut, olive, flax, hempseed, avocado, and red palm
- Small quantities of Himalayan salt, Celtic salt, raw honey, pure maple syrup, date sugar, and coconut sugar

And the most important ingredient of all: *love.*

Let's talk about fruit and why it should be an important staple in your pet's diet.

First, fruit is considered the food with the highest quantity of good bacteria. Friendly bacteria is necessary for the survival of hydrochloric acid, which is critical for proper digestion and assimilation. A healthy gut means a healthy immune system. In the stomachs of healthy humans, there are approximately seven different acids that make up the acidic environment of the gut. Dogs and cats have their own blend, made up of twenty different acids. This is one way we are biologically different from the animal species.

Although we are different, fruit contains an essential number of disease-fighting bacteria that greatly assist in restoring the healthy acids in the stomach that are necessary for the overall well-being of both humans and animals. Fruit consumption can prevent and discontinue most abnormal growths, which include lipomas, a common lump under the skin that many dogs and cats develop due to eating the nutrient-depleted and highly processed modern pet diets. Daily fruit consumption can also assist in the prevention of different types of pet cancers. The high antioxidant content in fruits will greatly support your pet's immune system, their first line of defense against disease.

What About Carbs and Sugar?

All carbohydrates are not the same. Removing the processed, modern *carbs*—also known as products made with white flour and or modern wheat—is wise because they don't exist in nature and are not recognized by the body. Consumption of these carbs can pose many health issues in both humans and animals as they deplete the body of vital nutrition. Furthermore, you and your pet need carbohydrates in the right form.

The Importance of Fruit

What is a carbohydrate? *Carb* means fiber and *hydrate* means water. If you have a fruit fear, avoiding this highly nutritious food because of its sugar content, your cells will most likely dehydrate—and this applies to your dog or your cat as well.

Your four-legged furry friend needs fruit for:

- Healthy skin
- Healthy detoxification
- A healthy brain and nervous system
- Optimal energy
- To be free of allergies
- Joint health
- Immune system support
- Presence of good bacteria critical for survival

The body heals on glucose because the body runs on glucose. The brain in both humans and animals is about 80 percent glucose and needs glucose in order to function. The brain converts glucose into glycogen for healthy memory and concentration. Keep in mind, the brain controls every organ system in the body, which means we need to fuel it properly.

This form of glucose is not the same as sugar from the sugar bowl, which can be harmful to your and your pet's health. Fruit sugar is the medicinal glucose fuel the body runs on. These forms of sugars are called *polysaccharides*, or complex carbohydrates. The high fiber content in fruit slows down the glycemic delivery because it must be digested.

Please know this: Fruit was the first food in the Garden of Eden and was the biggest staple in the diet of humans and animals alike. Fruit contains the highest amounts of biotics, the most important form of life force on planet Earth.

If you or your animal are eating better but still are not eating enough fruit because you're in fear of the *sugar,* then remember this: Fruit sugars known as polysaccharides are processed much differently in the body than processed sugar from the sugar bowl.

The infinite wisdom of the body knows the difference. When your pet doesn't eat enough fruit, their body will not absorb the nutrients in other food efficiently. *Why?* Because your pet needs the biotics in fruit in order to absorb, assimilate, metabolize, and utilize them properly. Otherwise, health issues will arise over time, and your pet will not heal optimally and fully.

How Much Fruit Per Day?

There's really no limit on fruit intake for your furry buddy; however, approximately ½ cup of 2–3 types of each fruit per day is sufficient. Adjust according to the appetite and size of your furry friend.

What About Protein?

Protein is a chain of amino acids essential in every living thing. It is the building block of all life mass. Protein is naturally occurring and present in everything you consume. We couldn't avoid it if we tried.

Animals and humans alike could never be lacking or deficient in protein. Now with all foods naturally containing protein, please do understand that all meats and eggs are considered *complete proteins* since they are the only foods that do not contain carbohydrates and are primarily protein.

In both animals and humans, a diet consisting of only or mostly protein sources—meat and eggs—can result in serious health issues.

When preparing your pet's meals, please do keep in mind that they are allowed to have most fruits and vegetables and be creative with that versatility. There's no actual recipe; just have fun using these principles and guidelines. Some of my top suggestions of the most beneficial produce for your furry friends are: sweet potatoes, pumpkin, carrots, bananas, pears, papaya, mangos, watermelon, apples, and berries—especially wild blueberries, which can easily be found frozen and can be defrosted before serving.

Considering the lists above, each meal should consist of a starch such as pumpkin or potato, a meat source, and a green vegetable. You may alternate with a grain or add a grain along with the meal, a few times per week. Each ingredient should be of equal parts to the others. Cooking oils for sautéing should be about one tablespoon per each pound of meat source. If you're adding vegetables, then you'll need to increase the oil by one teaspoon per cup.

Making meals in advance and storing them in plastic containers in the freezer is a wise choice. You can store meals in the freezer for up to four months. Please never use the microwave to defrost or cook your pet's meals. If you've read the chapter titled "What's Cooking America" in my first book, *STOP Battling Disease & Start Building Wellness: Your Guide to Extraordinary Health,* then you already know the detrimental effects of microwave usage.

Always be sure to use organically sourced ingredients for optimal flavor, a much-lessened toxic overload of chemical fertilizers, and the highest in nutritional value.

VEGAN PET DIETS

A vegan-based diet can be extremely beneficial for your pet if you're trying to reverse a current illness or are just implementing it periodically for cleansing. I would not suggest vegan diets for cats and dogs as a long-term lifestyle. Although many animals are plant eaters, I do believe that dogs and cats need animal protein. If you are adamant about a vegan diet for your pet, please do supplement with a good fish oil, which I will discuss in Chapter Three.

HEALTHY FOOD HABITS

A healthy diet for your dog and cat is critical for optimal health and can make a huge difference in the prevention and the reversal of many health issues your pet may be currently experiencing. Do keep in mind that most commercial dog foods are full of hormones, antibiotics, and sewer sludge and are topped with synthetic vitamins that cause more harm. Even though organic kibble is a better choice, it is still extruded at very high temperatures that destroy the goodness of real food.

Some companies provide higher quality foods than others, but I recommend minimizing the amount of commercial food you feed your pets.

Here are my top suggestions for commercially prepared dog and cat foods:

1. *The Honest Kitchen*
2. *K9 Granola Factory foods and treats*
3. *Castor & Pollux Organix canned and dry foods and treats*
4. *Newman's Own foods and treats*

5. *Signature Instinct frozen, raw food, and kibble*
6. *Nummy Tum Tum: Organic Canned Pumpkin, Apple, Berry Lovin, and Sweet Potato*

In my professional opinion, homemade pet food is best simply because you have control over the freshness and quality of ingredients. Here are a few simple, sample meal suggestions for your loving pets that you can make right at home:

Grass-fed ground beef sautéed in extra virgin coconut oil, organic peas and carrots—frozen is fine—sprouted rolled oats, sweet potatoes, and a pinch of Himalayan salt and served with love.

Sautéed pastured, boneless chicken in coconut oil, zucchini, red and yellow peppers, peas, topped with hemp seeds and served with love.

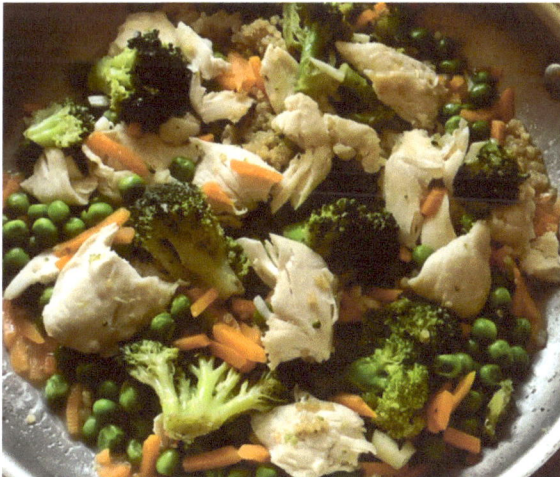

Sautéed Chicken with Veggies

I suggest that you give your pet a vegetarian meal at least twice per week such as:

- Oatmeal or quinoa with berries
- Mixed veggies
- Any suggested grain
- Pumpkin
- Red skin or sweet potatoes
- All fruit

This is a great way to allow the body to rest and not overwork the digestion process.

What About Treats and Snacks?

I personally give my dogs raw carrots for treats, and boy oh boy, do they love them. In addition, apples, raw celery, cucumbers, raw string beans, raw snap peas, and raw zucchini make for great crunchy snacks in lieu of processed treats—and they won't pack on unwanted pounds. My top suggestions in the list above for the better varieties of commercially prepared foods and treats can also be added in moderation.

I find that a lot of pet owners give their fur-babies peanut butter. If you've read my first two books, you'll have learned that modern peanuts, even organic, have aflatoxins or mycotoxins. These are carcinogenic—cancer-causing—compounds. They are not found in the wild peanut but do exist in the modern peanut. These toxins also are responsible for the high rate of peanut allergy issues in most children today.

Jungle peanuts are the original, wild peanuts that do not contain these toxins, making them perfectly safe and highly nutritious. In my cookbook, I substitute wild jungle peanut butter for modern peanut butter. In honor of my beloved golden retriever Peanut and his brother Milky Way, I put together a delicious, healthy, pet-friendly treat that your pets will absolutely love.

P.S. I eat them too. LOL

Peanut & Milky Way Treats

You will need:

1 tablespoon extra-virgin coconut oil

12 medjool dates, pits removed

¼ cup plus 1 tablespoon full fat coconut milk

½ cup oat flour

4 tablespoons of jungle peanut butter

Instructions:

Add all ingredients to a food processor or a high-speed blender and blend for 1–2 minutes or until everything is combined. Roll batter into 1-inch balls and place on parchment paper and freeze for two hours. Remove from the freezer, and you and your four-legged friend are ready to eat.

These delicious treats can be stored in an airtight container in the refrigerator for up to two weeks.

Why Our Furry Friends Eat Grass

Grass consumption is totally healthy and wise because your pet knows exactly when he or she needs a cleanse or a fiber boost. It does not necessarily indicate sickness. If your pet is excessively eating grass and other natural forages, then it may be time for a visit to the vet.

Let's take a look at how much food to give your dog or cat depending on their size. These amounts give you the total that is recommended for your pet over a 24–hour time period. Most adult dogs and cats should eat two meals per day, whereas puppies and kittens require three or more feedings.

As far as my suggestions for prepackaged foods, please follow the suggested amounts stated on the package.

HOMEMADE FOOD DAILY MEASUREMENTS FOR DOGS AND CATS

Pet Weight	Serving Size
3–12 lb.	⅓–1 cup
13–20 lb.	1–1⅓ cups
21–35 lb.	1⅓–2 cups
36–50 lb.	2–2⅔ cups
51–75 lb.	2⅔–3⅓ cups
76–100 lb.	3⅓–4¼ cups
Over 100 lb.	4¼ cups plus ¼ cup for each additional 10 lb. of body weight over 100 lb.

Please note that this is a standard guideline only. Specific bio-individual needs for your pet will vary depending on their personal requirements. Therefore, it is always best to check with your veterinarian.

WHAT ABOUT RAW MEAT FOR OUR FURRY FRIENDS?

We are really starting to see the rise of raw food diets in both animals as well as humans, and many pet food companies are adding raw ingredients to their formulas. Raw foods are much higher in enzymes, which are super important for optimal digestion. These foods are very minimally processed, leaving all vital nutrients intact.

If you are considering or already incorporate a raw food diet for your four-legged friend, please be sure to choose *organic* and *grass-fed* options to avoid harmful bacteria that are found in factory-farmed foods.

WHAT ABOUT MARROW BONES?

I highly suggest marrow bones for your fur baby because they are loaded with minerals that are excellent for both dogs and cats.

The high mineral content inside marrow bones can make a positive impact on the health of your pet. The minerals are extremely beneficial for their teeth and keep your pet's breath fresh. If you choose to give your pets raw meaty bones, start slow by only allowing them to chew for about fifteen minutes a day. You can gradually increase the amount of time by adding five minutes per day until their bodies get used to it. Do not exceed one half hour in total per day, as this may result in loose stools.

Please, never feed your pet cooked bones because they can splinter in your pet's intestines and cause a host of problems. In addition, they cannot be digested properly.

If you can find a local farm that practices humane, grass-fed farming methods, this will be your best choice.

THE CAT AND THE RAT

Although a cat chasing a mouse or a rat may be considered as a natural activity, eating rodents can pose great health risks to your beloved feline. These issues may include: rat poisoning, intestinal worms, or *toxoplasmosis*, a condition caused by undercooked meat, cat feces, or consumption of rats, in addition to other serious infections that could all result in death. If in the event you detect that your cat has eaten a rat and is showing unusual symptoms, I suggest you immediately take them to the vet.

ALLERGIES AND SKIN ISSUES

So many pet owners are misled into allergy testing. I don't agree with these tests simply because we are not allergic to real, whole, unprocessed, God-made food. What you and your furry companion may really be allergic to is *what's been done to the food.* Our foods may be impacted by pesticides, genetically engineered organisms, artificial ingredients, growth hormones, toxic vaccinations, prescription drugs, pasteurization, and on and on. You may be frustrated after trying every pet food out there without seeing any positive changes in your pet's health, and this may be the reason: *it may be all about what has been done to the food your pet is eating.*

Many people will come home from a vet appointment as if they've received the winning lottery numbers. Based on their allergy test, they now have a list of foods their furry friend should avoid. These foods may not even be the culprit; in fact, they may very well be some of the exact foods that lead to healing. Often, these same foods that are free of the allergy-related chemical cocktails should not be excluded from your pet's diet. In my professional opinion, allergy testing serves as a false answer to your pet's symptoms.

Regardless of which of my dietary suggestions you choose for your pet, I can guarantee that you will see tremendous positive changes in their health. When implementing the principles stated in this book, be creative and have fun. Great health and healing doesn't have to be confusing and stressful. We actually just need to go back to the simplicity of nature.

Testimonials

Here are two testimonials from pet patients that have made my simple dietary changes:

Buggles' Testimony, *written by his owner/daddy, Joe Lemoine*

Tonijean, it's funny how you were my third choice when it came to getting care for my dog, Buggles, but obviously God saved the best for last.

Buggles, my nine-year-old pug/Boston terrier, started having occasional seizures when she was two years old. As the years passed, the frequency of her seizures increased, and as of this past November, were coming consistently every five days. Going to our vet, she was put on seizure meds, which sadly made them even more frequent. Believing she was dying, I fasted and prayed and felt led to bring her to a holistic vet. She was taken off the meds and her regular diet of Pedigree dry dog food (with some meat) and put on a high fat keto diet (fatty meat with lots of fat). Surprisingly, the seizures stopped and I was so grateful, but, unfortunately, her health and quality of life took a turn for the worse. She went from weighing 24 pounds to 27 pounds in two months and couldn't even jump up into my lap. She became clumsy, falling over when I'd give a little pull on her leash. Our walks decreased from over two miles to one as she had little to no energy. She became congested almost immediately and after numerous calls and visits to the holistic vet, nothing changed. Lastly, she no longer had regular bowel movements, or urination for that matter, and her breaking wind was disgusting and putrid.

With my wife's encouragement from her personal experience with your services, I contacted you and set up an appointment. Following your nutritional outline to the 'T,' she is doing so well. She eats everything on her diet including the snacks. She has energy, she's lost weight, she's no longer congested or clumsy, her bowel movements are normal, and she looks great. And best of all, she now hasn't had a seizure in over five months.

Words can't express how grateful I am to the Lord for giving me back my dog, Buggles. May God continue to use you mightily for His glory as you help others with their pets' health.

God bless,

Joe Lemoine

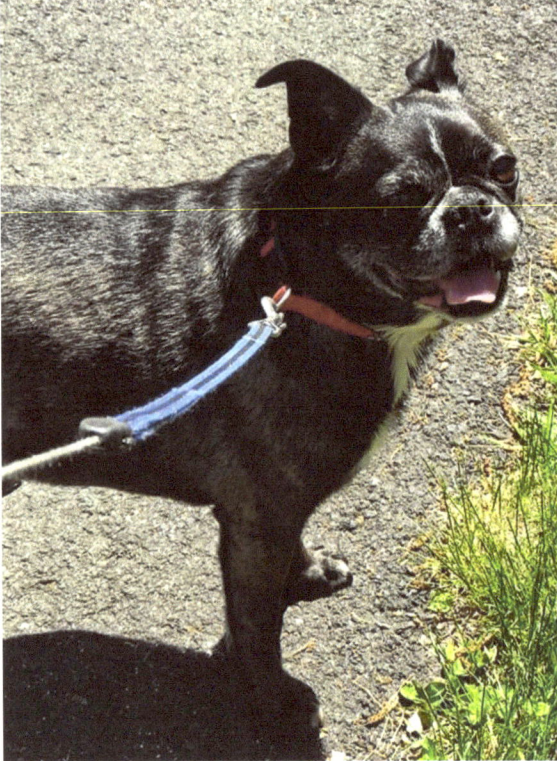

Buggles the Dog

The testimony of Mia, the beautiful Saint Bernard, follows. Mia has only had one appointment so far with me. When you diligently follow my God-given protocol, these are the results you can get after only five weeks.

Mia's Testimony

Tonijean! I just wanted to say hi and give you a Mia update. She is doing so unbelievably well. Her limp is COMPLETELY gone and her coat is so soft and shiny. She also has so much energy and we're going on at least 2+ hours of walks per day. The stairs are no longer a problem for her, and she runs up them!! I can't thank you enough for all your help and dedication to make sure she had the right supplements for optimal function. I know the turmeric, kelp, and flaxseed in addition to the other supplements and dietary changes are greatly helping. Thank you so much, Tonijean, for being such a bright light in my life. I truly appreciate your heart and spirit!. God Bless!

Lucia Albero

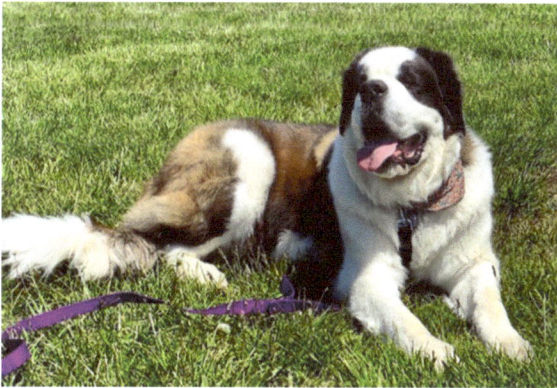

Mia the Dog

Thank you for completing Chapter Two because a healthy pet is a happy pet. My top food and treat suggestions can be found in the resource section of this book.

Chapter Three

Supplements

The wild-crafted medicines—which have always been on Planet Earth—are now called *supplements* in the modern world. Believe it or not, supplements have been consumed from the inception of time. The difference is that when we were hunter-gatherers, we literally went out into the wild and gathered them. Although we often don't think of our supplements this way, keep in mind that they are actually *foods*.

FOOD AS MEDICINE

Nowadays, we can purchase these exact nature-made supplements in health food stores or online. As far as recommendations for your four-legged friends, they should be based on the specific needs of each pet. The same goes for humans as well. However, I do suggest the following supplements as great additions to your pet's daily regimen. Please, always start out with less and gradually work your way up to a larger amount so your furry buddy can adapt gracefully. You should always follow the suggestions on the container or as prescribed by your pet's veterinarian for a more specific dosage based on your pooch's or kitty's needs.

Let's begin with probiotics because good bacteria, as you now know from Chapter Two, is critical for overall health. *Pro* means *for* and *bio* means *life*. A probiotic, therefore, could be described as a food that supports a healthy life. A daily dosage of a good probiotic can assure you that your pet is receiving a healthy balance of friendly gut flora.

I highly suggest *Mary Ruth's* pet probiotics because they are whole food and organic, exactly the way nature intended. Pet probiotics for dogs and cats are two separate formulas for optimizing the health of dogs and cats. I also love *Zesty Paws Probiotic Bites.* Probiotics can help rid the body of bad bacteria by colonizing the intestines. This will eliminate gas, keep your pet regular, and give their immune system the probiotic boost it so desperately needs.

BAD BREATH, TEETH, AND GUM HEALTH

A healthy gut also means a healthy mouth. I often see dogs and cats that suffer from bad breath and teeth and gum issues; I wholeheartedly believe it's their diet. As soon as they make dietary changes and augment with the right whole-food supplements, these conditions almost immediately disappear. Manufactured foods may be at the root of dental problems. Wild animals never go to the vet for a routine tooth cleaning, but their food source is certainly not coming from your local pet store.

There may be no need for routine dental appointments for your kitty and pooch if they have a healthy diet. Routine cleanings can destroy naturally occurring good bacteria necessary for fresh breath and healthy teeth and gums. However, if your vet feels it's necessary for your pet to have a cleaning due to a current issue, you absolutely need to pursue this.

SUPERFOODS FOR YOUR FUR-BABIES

In addition to probiotics, I also give Milky Way a regular dosage of *superfoods* and suggest you do as well.

Some excellent superfoods for pets are:

- Golden flax meal
- Medicinal mushrooms

- Spirulina
- Kelp
- Turmeric
- Barley grass juice

Bob's Red Mill Golden Flax Meal is a wonderful, fiber-rich, omega-3 superfood. It's great for its high nutrient and mineral content and adds the perfect flavor sprinkled over your pet's food. It's sure to please their palate.

Suggested Golden Flax Meal Dosage	
For dogs or cats	
1 teaspoon	15 lb. or less
½ tablespoon	16–25 lb.
1 tablespoon	26–55 lb.
1½ tablespoons	56 lb. and over

Increase a half tablespoon for every additional 10 lb.

Adding the right supplementation to your pet's diet can make such a tremendous impact on their current and future health. This is exactly why I suggest only specific brands that contain the highest quality of ingredients.

Medicinal mushrooms are some of nature's most powerful antidotes against cancer and other serious health issues. These nutritional powerhouses contain a myriad of anti-disease compounds. Their usage dates back thousands of years ago.

Milky Way loves *Zesty Paws;* therefore, I recommend *Zesty Paws Mushroom Bites.* They are packed with fourteen organic medical mushrooms that satisfy your pet's nutritional needs for this critical superfood: Organic Mushroom Blend (organic reishi, organic cordyceps, organic chaga, organic mesima, organic lion's mane, organic turkey tail, organic maitake, organic shiitake, organic blazei, organic poria, organic agarikon, organic suehirotake, organic oyster mushroom, organic true tinder polypore). You and I can feel happy about giving them to our furry loved ones.

Sea veggies, such as spirulina and kelp, are also super important to ensure optimal well-being for your cats and dogs. I recommend *Zesty Paws Superfood Bites,* another addition to my furry boy's daily regimen. This product contains both spirulina and kelp.

I like to call spirulina *plant blood* for its rich green color provided by chlorophyll. It detoxifies the body as soon as it's taken. What I love most about spirulina is its immune-boosting abilities. Spirulina increases the production of antibodies and activates killer T cells. Adding spirulina to your pet's daily diet can ward off toxicity in the blood, increase energy, and aid in the prevention of cancer and other debilitating conditions.

Kelp is another important sea vegetable that has the unique ability to increase activity in the thyroid, pituitary, and adrenal glands. The iodine content of kelp is phenomenal for thyroid conditions; iodine deficiencies are often seen in animal and human patients suffering from a malfunctioning thyroid.

It's truly amazing how nature itself is our best physician. God knows best, so He put medicine we all need right in the food:

And God said, "Behold, I have given you every herb-bearing seed which is upon the face of all the earth and every tree in the which is the fruit of a tree yielding seed; to you it shall be for food."

Genesis 1:29 (KJV)

As you now know, I love the quality of *Zesty Paws* products and, therefore, I highly recommend their multivitamins for their whole-food ingredients. I am also a huge fan of turmeric, and I recommend it to all my human and non-human patients for its incredible anti-cancer and anti-inflammatory properties. In addition, turmeric is great for optimizing brain function, supports healthy bones and joints, and is another food that contains good bacteria.

If you're looking for a powdered turmeric that you can sprinkle on your pet's food, I suggest an organic turmeric powder. Two of my top suggestions are *Terrasoul Superfoods Turmeric Powder and Navitas Turmeric Powder.*

Suggested Dosages for Terrasoul Superfoods and Navitas Turmeric Powder	
For dogs or cats	
⅛ teaspoon	15 lb. or less
½ teaspoon	16–25 lb.
1 teaspoon	26–55 lb.
1⅛ teaspoons	56 lb. and over

Increase ⅛ teaspoon for every additional 10 lb.

Barley grass juice powder is another one of my favorite superfoods. This green super-healing food improves skin health by cleansing the body of toxic heavy metals. It promotes bone and teeth health and has powerful antioxidant properties that boost immune system function up to 70 percent. Barley grass juice also helps heal fatty or sluggish liver by increasing bile, a critical fluid that helps your four-legged friend digest optimally.

Terrasoul also carries one of the best barley grass juice powders on the market. *Vimergy* is another excellent source for barley grass juice powder.

Suggested Dosage for Terrasoul and Vimergy Barley Grass Juice Powder	
For dogs or cats	
⅛ teaspoon	15 lb. or less
½ teaspoon	16–25 lb.
1 teaspoon	26–55 lb.
1⅛ teaspoons	56 lb. and over

Increase ⅛ teaspoon for every additional 10 lb.

Good Old Vitamin C

Let's take a look at vitamin C. Real whole-food vitamin C is necessary for the repair of all bodily tissues. Keep in mind that ascorbic acid is a synthetic form of vitamin C and is not found in nature. Please refer to the chapter titled "The Truth About Supplements" in my first book, *Stop Battling Disease & Start Building Wellness*. This artificial form of so-called vitamin C can be toxic to your pet's health, as well as yours. Real vitamin C has a high antioxidant content, making this nutrient an important weapon in strengthening the function of the immune system. Vitamin C works synergistically with other nutrients in helping the body optimize assimilation and absorbability. It is also extremely beneficial to combat colds and infections, enhance wound healing, and strengthen bones and teeth. Vitamin C is important for healthy blood flow, which helps your furry friend maintain a shiny, sleek coat.

My top suggestions for the best sources of vitamin C are *Garden of Life Raw Vitamin C* and *Nutrigold Vitamin C Gold*. They are provided in the form of capsules that can be opened and added directly to your pet's food.

Suggested Dosages for Garden of Life Raw and Nutrigold Vitamin C Gold Capsules	
For dogs or cats	
½ capsule	15 lb. or less
1 full capsule	16–25 lb.
1½ capsules	26–55 lb.
2 capsules	56 lb. and over

Increase a half capsule for every additional 10 lb.

WHAT ABOUT FISH OIL?

What about fish oil, you ask? First and foremost, when looking for a good fish oil, you must be sure it's wild. Now if you've read my first book, then you'll remember the chapter titled "Farmed and Dangerous."

Just to simplify, farmed fish is definitely a big NO since these fish swim in cesspools of their own fecal matter. They are fed a diet of artificial pellets, making their flesh and oil unhealthy and toxic. Wild fish, on the other hand, are eating their natural diet of omega-rich sea plants or other fish that eat the same.

Fish oil is extremely healthy for both your kitty and doggie. Whether you choose cod liver oil or salmon oil, just be sure the source is wild. Wild fish oil is loaded with omega 3, which increases mobility in joints, enhances strong bones and teeth, protects the brain and central nervous system, supports heart health, keeps viruses out of the body, and is another immune-building supplement your best friend will surely benefit from.

Here are my top suggestions;

1. *Nordic Naturals Omega-3 Pet, Nordic Naturals Pet Cod Liver Oil*
2. *Zesty Paws Wild Alaskan Salmon Oil*
3. *Holistic Pet Organics Wild Deep Sea Salmon Oil*

Please follow the suggestions on the packaging based on your pet's size.

DEWORMING

Being a naturopath, I clearly did not want to use the typical chemical-laden dewormer, and of course, I didn't want my pup to suffer from worms. When my mom was a little girl, she told me that she never forgot how her parents—my grandparents—dewormed their first dog. Back then, it was popular to use straight, raw garlic. Yep, you read that right! She said, after several hours of their puppy eating the garlic, what looked like spaghetti to my mom came out of their furry baby.

This story, of course, remained in my mind. However, I've always known that garlic is a forbidden food for both dogs and cats. I realize it was used once on puppies for deworming and was considered safe. However, a component of garlic called *n-propyl disulfide* has the potential to cause anemia in dogs and cats. Fortunately, garlic is almost always prescribed for pets with parasites and is safe and effective in the correct dosage.

Here's the thing: you must not exceed five or more grams of garlic per kilo of body weight. To translate, one clove of garlic typically weighs between one and two grams; therefore, a medium-sized dog or cat would have to consume four cloves per day to become toxic.

With this said, as long as you're using garlic wisely, it can be beneficial for the reduction of worms and or other nasty critters infiltrating your furry buddy.

I decided it was a go for both of my boys, Peanut and Milky Way, in addition to an all-natural, safe, and effective product called *Pet Wellbeing GI Cleanup Gold* for dogs. They also have a *GI Cleanup* version for your feline. This strategy worked wonderfully for my dogs, and they've never had any issues since. I also recommend this to all my pet patients, and they have reaped the same great results.

Now, if you're not comfortable with using garlic from time to time, or doing a garlic deworming, please feel free to check with your veterinarian or look into the Pet Wellbeing products.

Suggested Garlic Dosages	
For dogs or cats	
3–12 lb.	1 clove garlic given each day for 3 days until results are achieved.
13–25 lb.	1½ cloves for 3 days as stated above.
Over 25 lb.	2 cloves for 3 days until results are achieved.

Side note: I personally love all Pet WellBeing products and highly recommend them.

A Brief Note on Pet Diarrhea

From time to time, you'll find that your four-legged friend will have a soft stool. Most of the time, this is not a concern. Our fur-babies will find and consume things they shouldn't be eating and their bodies will get rid of it. I always suggest slippery elm bark, an incredible herb with antimicrobial properties that effectively targets gastrointestinal issues. Organic Traditions is the brand I recommend. See below for dosage recommendations.

Dosages for Slippery Elm Bark (powdered form)	
For dogs and cats	
½ teaspoon	15 lb. and under
1 teaspoon	16–25 lb.

Add ½ teaspoon for every additional 15 lb.

In addition to slippery elm, you can give an increase of probiotics for a few days until symptoms disappear. Dogs and cats both do very well with a ½–1 teaspoon of raw honey right off the spoon, the amount depending on the size of your furry friend. Real, raw honey has excellent antimicrobial properties making it a great medicine for soothing an upset tummy, in addition to being great tasting.

Continual diarrhea and or other symptoms of concern may be a reason for a trip to your veterinarian for a more personalized checkup.

WHAT DOES HEALTHY PET POOP LOOK LIKE?

The average color of dog and cat stool should be chocolate or dark brown. You don't want a stool too dark, or black in color, as this could mean blood. If this occurs, Rover or Sylvester may need a visit to the vet. The size will vary depending on the size of your pet, but typically 1–3 inches in length, 1–2 inches in width, and about the shape of a tootsie roll sounds about right. Extra-large breeds could have a stool size as big as 5 inches long with a 2–3 inch width. With both dogs and cats, the consistency should be firm, but a little clay-like is perfectly normal.

If you or your pet are having health issues, please keep in mind that it's not so much about what to take to make the problem go away; it's more about removing the cause so the body can heal. Symptoms are the body's way of reacting to foreign invaders, such as chemical fertilizers, genetically engineered foods, artificial ingredients, vaccines, and prescription drugs.

Symptoms will not go away until the body doesn't have a reason to create symptoms anymore. Symptoms are messages letting you know something is wrong. We don't want to cover up the symptoms.

Thank you for reading Chapter Three because a healthy pet is a happy pet. My top suggestions for supplements can be found in the resource section of this book.

Chapter Four

Bath-time, Bug Repellant, and More

A healthy, shiny coat on your kitty and pooch definitely comes from within. Proper nutrition is the key to a healthy exterior, but you will also have to occasionally bathe and groom your furry friend.

BATH CARE

How often do I bathe my beautiful Milky Way, you ask? First, as soon as I say the word bath to Milky Way, I chase him around the house for an hour, just like I chased my beloved Peanut. After he surrenders, we lather up.

If you have a golden or another big dog, you know you're getting in that tub too. LOL

I believe the appropriate amount of time in between baths for your dog or cat is about a month. There is nothing like their own natural oils for keeping their skin and coat healthy. The oils work like medicine to keep skin and hair from getting itchy or dry. Your pet's skin also has a naturally protective microbiome, which is a population of friendly microorganisms. Over-washing can destroy these beneficial microbes, leaving their skin more at risk of infection.

Many of the commercial brands of pet care skin products are full of toxic chemicals that have the potential to cause serious health issues. Most of their ingredients never existed in nature; some may be highly carcinogenic. Therefore, usage over time can pose great health risks to your fur-babies.

Let's take a good look at some of the best and safest non-toxic products on the market for shampoos, conditioners, and bug repellents.

I absolutely love *EarthBath Totally Natural Pet Care* products and so will you. *Simply Pure Natural Pet Products* is another winner. The *Earth Animal* product line is another one of my favorites.

My suggestions will greatly help if your pet has itchy skin or skin allergies, although they should be on the mend since you're now following my nutritional guidelines in this book.

COCONUT OIL

Extra-virgin coconut oil is not only an excellent ingredient for your pet's diet; it can also do wonders for dry or itchy skin when applied topically. Even if your furry buddy doesn't have skin issues, applying coconut oil to their skin helps maintain moisture. Coconut oil is loaded with antimicrobial properties that starve the bad bacteria that might lead to future skin problems.

I suggest using any organic extra-virgin coconut oil that you would use for cooking; if it's good enough to eat, then it's good enough for your pet's skin. Remember, everything is absorbed through the skin.

Here are a few suggestions:

- *Nutiva Extra-Virgin Coconut Oil*
- *Dr. Bronner's Extra-Virgin Coconut Oil*
- *Garden of Life Raw Extra-Virgin Coconut Oil*

CLEANING YOUR PET'S EARS

Every time I would say the words, "Mama's gonna clean your ears," Peanut would run like his life depended on it and hide. Now, my Milky Way does the exact same thing. I really believe that Peanut spiritually tells his brother Milky Way to make a run for it when Mama mentions bath time or ear cleaning. LOL

Keeping your pets' ears clean is important to prevent yeast overgrowth that leads to ear mites and infections. I recommend cleaning once or twice a month, although the timeframe for cleanings will vary depending on your furry friend's breed, level of activity, amount of fur, wax production, and of course, their age.

Keeping it simple, I always use good old raw apple cider vinegar with H_2O. I take about 6 ounces of pure water and 3 ounces of raw apple cider vinegar and add to a dropper bottle. I then insert about one full dropper into each ear. Massage the base of the ear for 5–7 seconds and you're good to go. You can store this product for up to one year in your pet-friendly medicine cabinet.

I also love to use Bodhi ear cleaner for both pooches and kitty cats. It's 100 percent natural, safe, and effective, and it's made with raw apple cider vinegar. A healthy diet and supplements will also help keep your pet's body in optimal health, preventing unwanted ear issues. As a practitioner, I've discovered that pets with frequent ear problems are usually over-vaccinated and overmedicated, and they have a poor-quality diet. Always keep in mind that great overall health starts from within.

How to Trim Your Pet's Nails Safely

Peanut was actually wonderful when it came time for Daddy to give him his 3–4 week manicure and pedicure. Milky Way is getting better at having it done since I do believe that Peanut supernaturally lets him know he will survive the process.

Every 3–4 weeks is just about the perfect time for trimming your furry buddy's nails. Keeping an accurate schedule will help prevent overgrown nails, hangnails, and other unwanted nail problems.

1. Hold their paw steady and firmly.

2. Gently hold the nail at a 45-degree angle.

3. Snip off a small bit of the end of each nail, about ⅟₁₆ of an inch.

Be sure to strictly avoid the nerve, as cutting this will create bleeding and pain. *Never* put the entire nail into the clipper. For pets with white nails, you can easily see the pink part of the nail (the quick) that you need to avoid with your clipper. For pets with black nails, it is difficult to see the pink, but you will see a groove in the nail—that is the mark for you to stop trimming.

Keep in mind that pets that walk on hard surfaces don't require their mani-pedi as frequently.

If you're too afraid to take on the task of nail trimming, then by all means, go to a good groomer who will do the job for you. Always observe the process to avoid any unwanted issues with your groomer.

DECLAWING CATS

If you want my opinion on whether or not to have your cat declawed, then my answer would be *absolutely not*—but your final decision is up to you. Declawing your purr baby is inhumane and takes away their dignity, especially since kneading is a natural and common behavior of the domestic cat.

In my opinion, declawing is barbaric and cruel. It causes pain in their paws, risk of infection, body weakness, pain, and necrosis of the tissue, which means tissue death. Your purr baby was created perfectly just as they are by our loving God.

To keep a cat's claws from growing back—making this surgical procedure *successful*—part of their bone and nerve is removed. The removal of a cat's claws is similar to a human having the tip of their finger taken off. OUCH! It's also like that awful feeling when you're wear a pair of shoes that don't fit all day long.

Fur Brushing and Normal Shedding

How often should you brush your fur-baby?

Shorter-haired breeds of both dogs and cats usually do well with a good brushing about 1–2 times per week. Longer-haired cats and dogs like my golden need their locks brushed at least once per day. Brushing not only increases the natural oil production for a shiner coat, it also reduces shedding. I bet those of you who have longer-haired pets can relate to the daily vacuuming chore. Shedding is a normal occurrence in all types of breeds as this is a natural process just like with human hair. Humans lose anywhere from 80–100 hairs per day, whereas cats and dogs only shed twice per year, in spring and fall—although it seems like every day.

Daily shedding isn't actually shedding but a normal breakage of excess fur. Springtime shedding occurs when your pet's coat lightens up for the warmer weather, and autumn is when their coat sheds before being replaced with a thicker, warmer coat. From tons of experience, may I suggest that your vacuum cleaner is in top-notch shape during these two seasons.

Excessive Shedding

Excessive shedding or fur loss may be a reason for you to take your furry friend for a trip to the veterinarian for an evaluation.

Some possible underlying conditions that cause excessive shedding are:

- Parasites (fleas, mites, or lice)
- Thyroid or adrenal malfunction
- Toxic-food-related issues

- Infections
- Allergic reactions to oral or topical medications

BUG REPELLENT

Keeping the pests away from your fur baby can be tough since most commercial bug repellents are full of toxic ingredients known to cause cancer and other serious health issues. Well, no need to look any further because *Earth Animal* makes a wonderful product called *Dr. Bob Goldstein's Natural Protection Herbal Bug Spray.* This product safely keeps fleas, ticks, and even mosquitoes far away from your fur-babies. *Greener Organic Ways Bug Repellent* is another one of my top suggestions.

TICK BITE

If you suspect your pet has been bit by a tick, feel around their fur until you find the tick. Removing the tick with a tip tweezer by separating the fur and lifting the tick from the base is best for total removal. Do not twist or turn the tweezer since this will result in parts of the tick remaining behind. It's best to remove the tick as soon as possible since it takes twenty-four hours for transmission of disease. Another option is to to drown the tick with petroleum jelly or rubbing alcohol while on your pet and then removing it the same way with tweezers—or it may just fall off.

If you are concerned your pet may have contracted a tick-borne illness, then please take them to their veterinarian for further observations.

A healthy diet, whole food supplementation, nontoxic body care, and lots of love are all the ingredients you'll need to give your furry family members a long and healthy life.

They went into the ark with Noah, two and two of all flesh in which there was the breath of life.

Genesis 7:15 (ESV)

Thank you for reading Chapter Four because a healthy pet is a happy pet. My top suggestions for products mentioned in this chapter can be found in the resource section of this book.

Chapter Five

Neutering, Spaying, and Vaccinations

Many pet owners have been called irresponsible for not neutering and spaying their pets. There's a lot of financial gain behind this scare tactic to get you, the pet owner, to follow through. I have seen pets spayed and neutered as early as three months of age. The truth is, a responsible pet owner will not allow their un-neutered or un-spayed pet to roam freely and breed with other dogs or cats.

Another fear tactic used to get you to spay and neuter is the threat of ovarian, cervical, or testicular cancers. In my professional opinion, this is no different than an oncologist suggesting you have your child's breast, ovaries, and uterus removed to prevent cancer or to recommend the castration of young boys to prevent prostate problems as an adult.

Ever Wonder Why There's Such an Increase in Pet Cancers?

Spaying and neutering puts your pet at great risk of many types of cancers and other debilitating diseases. Hormones work as antioxidants in the body; they assist in the fight against cancer and other health problems.

Neutering and spaying increases the risk of many health issues with your pet. Your pet's reproductive system produces these important hormones, which are critical for the healthy development of bones and ligaments. If these hormones are removed, especially too early, they won't have enough time to complete their job.

Neutering and spaying does not prevent testicular, prostate, and ovarian cancers as you've been told. If anything, according to these facts, the effects are the complete opposite.

According to a Rutgers University study, if spaying or neutering is done before one year of age, your dog or cat will most likely have:

1. Increased risk of splenic hemangiosarcoma

2. Significantly increased risk of bone cancer (osteosarcoma)

3. Increased risk of obesity

4. Tripled risk of hypothyroidism

5. Increased risk of recurrent urinary tract infections, recessed vulva, vaginal dermatitis, vaginitis, and doubled risk of urinary tract tumors. Urinary tract issues, including spay incontinence, occur in 4–20 percent of dogs.

6. Increased risk of orthopedic disorders, including hip and elbow dysplasia

7. Increased risk of adverse reactions to vaccinations[1]

The Importance of Hormones

The hormone system in both male and female dogs and felines takes two complete years to fully develop. Female dogs and cats typically get their menstrual cycle around the age of six months, so early spaying keeps this normal, natural process from ever occurring.

Hormones are absolutely vital for the full development of the feminine and masculine features of your dog and cat. Having your pet neutered

---

1 Sanborn, Laura. "Long-Term Health Risks and Benefits Associated with Spay/Neuter in Dogs." *National Animal Interest Alliance.* 14 May 2007. www. naiaonline.org/pdfs/LongTermHealthEffectsOfSpayNeuterInDogs.pdf

or spayed, especially before the age of two years of age, inhibits proper growth potential, heightens their risk of serious health issues, and will affect their overall appearance.

As a practitioner, I have seen countless cats and dogs who have suffered from various health conditions as a result of spaying or neutering. In a neutered male, the head and chest are not as broad as they are in a male that's un-neutered. Females experience recurrent urinary tract infections and a laundry list of other health issues. Early-neutered males and early-spayed females seem to be taller and lankier than pets whose owners waited until they were fully developed. Female and male pets that are not neutered or spayed early have more distinct feminine and masculine appearances overall. Think about it. These invasive procedures are basically de-sexing your pet and are one of the top contributors to many pet health issues.

If you choose to have your pet spayed or neutered, please wait until they are at least two years of age to avoid some of these serious health concerns.

SAFER ALTERNATIVES

Another much safer alternative is to find a veterinarian who will perform a vasectomy in males or a tubal ligation for females—also known as having the tubes tied. The reason this less invasive procedure is not commonly recommended is simply because it's not as profitable.

For the love of money is the root of all evil: which while some coveted after, they have erred from the faith, and pierced themselves through with many sorrows.

1 Timothy 6:10 (KJV)

Vaccinations: A Medical Timebomb

As a professional with a brain, I do understand why people are afraid and rely on vaccination as a means of disease prevention, and I highly respect each of you who feel this way. You are being cautious, and this is how you've been taught—that vaccines have saved and will save lives. You also feel that anyone who doesn't vaccinate themselves or their pets must be crazy and irresponsible.

But please, read on . . .

In my professional opinion, the theory behind original vaccines made sense. They were used to prevent disease by using an arm-to-arm method of inoculation of the species from the infected person in the hope of creating an immune response and building antibodies against the disease. This is exactly what the infinite wisdom of the immune system was designed to do.

As a naturopathic, drugless, holistic practitioner, I know firsthand that nature provides everything we need not only to prevent all forms of sickness but also to provide healing in the event a person has a health condition. Nature's pharmacy provides exactly what works best in sync with our natural defenses. I've worked with countless human and animal patients to completely reverse many so-called incurable diseases, where the medical establishment has failed greatly.

Fortunately, both humans and animals were created to work in sync with nature as nature was created to work in sync with us. God has provided numerous natural remedies for natural immunization. The word *immunized* means that the immune system has detected an invader and—*naturally*, not *forcefully*—has done its job by creating killer T cells, cytotoxins, immunoglobulins, or lymphocytes to combat the invader.

This natural immunization process is corrupted by the presence of heavy metals from vaccines, which compromise your natural defenses, as well as your pet's. This is exactly why modern vaccinations are detrimental to the health of the recipient and may result in a host of other serious health issues.

Here's why—

Today's vaccine cocktails not only contain the disease, but they are also loaded with toxic ingredients, like heavy metals, that break down your natural defenses, poisoning your blood.

Here are some of the vaccine ingredients, just to name a few:

- Thimerosal
- Aluminum
- Formaldehyde
- Gelatin
- Yeast protein
- Antibiotics
- Egg protein
- Monosodium glutamate (MSG)
- Squalene
- Unrelated DNA and RNA
- Adjuvants—which shock your immune system
- Polysorbate 80
- Aborted human fetal tissue

You cannot expect a healthy immune response when pumping toxic poison into the blood of a human or animal; it's completely impossible. As a naturopath, I have worked successfully with many patients to reverse the horrific immunocompromising effects of these modern-day toxic drug injections. We cannot deny the number of artificially immunized and damaged victims in today's modern world. I see them firsthand as a practitioner. Human parents, including pet parents, live this nightmare each and every day of their lives because of their once-blind trust in the medical community. Modern vaccines with toxic ingredients do not *immunize*, they *compromise* and destroy lives.

Unfortunately, BIG pHARMa cannot patent nature and make their zillions of dollars from nature-made inoculations, from natural sources. Therefore, they concoct these toxic compounds made in a lab and use us—you, me, and our furry loved ones—as laboratory rats. They are also clever about using fear tactics to frighten you into believing that you will die without a vaccine and that nature cannot protect you.

So called immunology experts fail to tell you the horrific effects of the Standard American Diet (SAD) of microwaved and processed foods, foods that contain chemical fertilizers, genetically engineered food, pasteurized dead dairy, and hormone-laden, drugged-up meats—which include most commercially processed pet foods. All these food sources may be helping to destroy our natural defenses.

In its infinite wisdom, the immune systems of both humans and animals know exactly how to create antibodies against a disease naturally, without having to resort to the artificial, forced immunity from vaccination.

Artificial *immunity* through vaccination does not confer the same immunity that natural immunity to a disease does; in addition, it may result in overactivity and dysfunction of the immune system.

Natural immunity gives lifetime immunity whereas, even if a toxic drug injection works, the shelf life of the immunity is short-lived because vaccines work against the natural demeanor of the immune system.

There are detrimental effects of mass inoculating our pets; it creates vaccine resistance due to gene cell death and mutation of the disease. When you use an artificial means of immunity like vaccines, viruses and bacteria can mutate and multiply. This is the universal principle of all living things. Wherever you place a lab-altered form of so-called immunity, that organism is going to fight for survival, especially when the natural defenses have been altered through these toxic drug injections.

The immune system naturally detects an intruder, creating immunoglobulins to naturally eradicate the disease. The immune system will also produce killer T cells that recognize and eliminate any infected cells. This is called real, robust immunity and is not achieved through mass inoculation. The complete opposite occurs through vaccination.

For example, when you have enough influenza circulating around in a population, the unvaccinated and healthy population achieves a herd immunity effect because enough people have experienced it. Now those people are naturally protected, and this confers immunity for others. The more we vaccinate, the more we create an altered immunity, resulting in continued disease warfare.

I have seen numerous, overly vaccinated pets need repeated visits to the vet. This certainly is not a coincidence, but a result of severely altering natural immunity.

The rise in pet asthma, allergies, ear infections, skin issues, thyroid problems, digestive disorders, chronic anxiety, seizures, and different types of cancers, may be the result of several factors, such as mass inoculations, early neutering and spaying, and poor diet.

Once again . . .

Nature provides everything we need to live well and disease free, but in today's modern BIG pHARMa world, it's not profitable!

The *Vaccine Injury Compensation Act* has paid out billions of dollars to immunized and damaged individuals over the last decade alone. See for yourself at hrsa.gov/vaccine-compensation/index.html.

I am not telling you not to have your pet vaccinated; however, as a practitioner, I do believe it is extremely important that you understand the truth behind vaccines so you can make your own informed decision. Your decision should be based the reality of truth, not the fear and scare tactics used by most medical doctors and veterinarians.

If you have a pet that's currently immunization-damaged or if you're still considering vaccinations, please be sure to implement the principles in this book so your fur-babies can heal and live the lives they were created to live.

One of my top suggestions for healing is *milk thistle*. Once again, nature provides everything we need. The liver in both animals and humans is our filtration system. When it's filled with years of toxic heavy metals from vaccines and chemical fertilizers, milk thistle can help with rejuvenation of the liver. If you've ever cleaned a filter on a swimming pool, you know how that pool water looks when the filter is clogged. If the filter needs cleaning, it will not work until it's clean. I'm sure you would not want to swim in that pool water.

I am a huge fan of *Pet Wellbeing Milk Thistle*. Please use as suggested on the labeling.

Thank you for reading Chapter Five because a healthy pet is a happy pet. Additional pet detox products from vaccinations can be found in the resource section of this book and should be used as directed and assisted by a licensed veterinarian.

Chapter Six

Toys, Exercise, and Playtime

I believe the greatest years of our pets' lives are when we're playing together with them. The best memories are built and the most laughter is expressed. Playtime is a time when you and your fur-baby get to connect on a fun and exciting level where you can be yourselves. Playing catch or rolling in the mud, swimming, or just those well-earned belly rubs bring both of you such moments of overwhelming joy. Another great benefit of playtime is that our furry loved ones also get their daily dose of exercise.

Playing is a great way to bond. Playtime with your pet brings forth a release of the feel-good hormones: oxytocin, dopamine, and serotonin. These hormones are prerequisites to locking in your love affair even deeper.

Although my believed Peanut is no longer physically here, I have so many wonderful memories of being with him, and most are the ones we created during playtime. I loved when he would swim and run out on the grass and roll all over to dry off. His look of happiness brought a lifetime of such joy to my heart.

Peanut loved it when I rubbed his belly, and he knew how excited I got when he let me know it was time for Mama to get the belly massage going. If I was in another room, I could hear him whimpering simply because he was letting me know that he was upside-down with his belly up, ready and waiting. Oh, how I loved these moments.

HOW MUCH EXERCISE DO OUR FUR-BABIES NEED?

There isn't really a one-size-fits-all answer to the question of how much exercise your dog or cat needs. Of course, exercise is important, but the answer is determined by the breed, current health status, and age. Puppies usually have a whole lot more energy, so much that you'll commonly see them literally running around rapidly in circles. I've witnessed my Milky Way do this on several occasions during which we needed to get out the way for survival!

On average, I'd say a good rule is approximately between one and two hours of exercise daily. In my professional opinion, I believe it's best to take smaller intervals of exercise throughout the day rather than one long one. This is only if your schedule permits; most people work and can only dedicate a part of the day to exercising their four-legged friend.

Have you ever heard of the expression *fat cat?* It sounds both funny and even cute, but it may not be too healthy. A lot of indoor cats get this label, so if you're an indoor cat owner, you may need to encourage your feline to be more active.

I recommend that your kitty has at least twenty-five minutes or more of exercise daily. As with dogs, I also feel it's best to combine a few longer periods of time and a few shorter periods, depending on your pet's ability.

Play toys are always an easier, more acceptable way to get your four-legged buddy to move more. If you have a pet that has grown lazy over time, it's wise for you to encourage them, through playing, to become more active. Not only will you be lengthening their lifespan, but you'll also be bonding your relationship.

LET'S LOOK AT TOYS

Many pet toys on the market today contain toxic materials that are potentially harmful to your pet if ingested. What upsets me most as a pet owner is these warnings are right on the labels. Why even bother to create such harmful items when they are to be given to an innocent animal? To me, this practice makes absolutely no sense.

If your dog or cat is a chewer like mine, then you've most likely have seen pieces missing off their toys. The question is, where did those missing parts end up?

As a naturopathic practitioner and an animal lover, I've done my research on the best, non-toxic toys for our furry family members.

West Paw has some of the best nontoxic toys. Whether your pet likes to play rough or just to play lightly, their toys are designed for their specific desires. West Paw toys are extremely versatile; some are for more aggressive pets, while others are made for fetching, chewing, and for those cuddling moments.

Planet Paw is another great, non-toxic alternative for safer pet toys.

WHAT ABOUT SWIMMING?

Swimming is an excellent and fun activity for your pet, especially if you have a golden retriever like mine, or any dog that loves water. Swimming is extremely healthy for their bones and ligaments since it has a lower impact on their joints while increasing blood flow from the movement. Swimming has multiple benefits as it provides a great cardiovascular workout while increasing muscle. It's also a wonderful way to have your furry companion burn off that extra energy.

It still makes me chuckle, though, thinking about how much my goldens love swimming yet hide as soon as they hear the word *bath*. LOL. Does this sound familiar to you too?

Thank you for reading Chapter Six because a healthy pet is a happy pet. My top toy suggestions can be found in the resource section of this book.

Chapter Seven

Proper Rest and Sleep

After all that fun and play, our furry friends get tired and need their rest. Proper rest and sleep is critical for all ages and is the time when the body repairs and rejuvenates. It can also be a great time for you to get some important tasks completed. Adequate amounts of sleep are extremely important in the development of the brain and nervous system in puppies and kittens.

How Much Should My Pet Sleep?

In general, most dogs and cats sleep 12–16 hours per day. Puppies and kittens can sleep up to 18 hours per day. These long sleep hours are normal for our furry loved ones and are absolutely no reason for concern. These extended sleep times are a sign of contentment and security. In the wild, dogs and cats alike both slept these same long hours. It is a sign of peace and safety. If your furry friend is anxious and or restless, this could be a sign of fear or lack of security. In the event this is an issue, you may need to be more attentive to him or her. Showing more affection can rapidly remedy this condition.

If there's a lot of arguing or tension in a home, animals are extremely intuitive and can pick up negative vibes that affect their emotional health. If your situation is unavoidable, showing them more love will offset the atmosphere, giving your pet peace of mind.

If you feel your pet is sleeping excessively, this may not be normal and as a result, you should take a trip to your veterinarian for an evaluation.

Certain diseases can cause your pet to sleep unusually long hours. Some known factors are also stress, age-related issues, over-activity, or even separation anxiety. Often, pets go to a doggie daycare while their owners are working, and we find that for some, it's best their pet just stays at home in their own environment rather than being in an unfamiliar place. Dogs especially—but cats also—adapt to a sense of smell and feel much more comfortable with their own senses. This does not only pertain to their blankets and toys, but also that familiar aroma of their human family. Remember, the famous line from *The Wizard of Oz: There's no place like home* brought Dorothy and Toto right back where they belonged.

What Kind of Bed Is Best for My Furry Friend?

This is another question that doesn't have a one-size-fits-all answer. Some dogs and cats like a hard, cold floor, whereas others may like a soft, cozy, warm bed. Others, like my Milky Way, may like both and switch off throughout the night, depending on the temperature of the room. You also must take into consideration the breed, size, and just like humans, the time of year. We all like more warmth in the colder months and cooler bedrooms in the hot, steamy summer. Your furry loved ones may also agree.

As to whether or not your pet should sleep with you—it is really up to you. As you can see, I'm not about the one-size-fits-all answer or repeating the recycled misinformation that's out there. When it comes to giving your pet a good night's rest, most answers are based on your pet and your relationship. Some pet owners live alone with their dog or cat as their only companion; therefore, they become best buddies and sleep may well require a furry cuddle.

I personally always loved to sleep with my beloved Peanut until he got too big for the bed. Now with my precious Milky Way, the issue is the same. My hubby and I are tall and we take up most of the bed. With a full-sized golden retriever added to the mix, it can be extremely uncomfortable and no one gets a good night's rest.

I've had this discussion with many pet owners and some jokingly say, "My husband can always sleep in the pet bed!"

Shhhh . . . I've also said this on many occasions. LOL. Have you?

The bottom line is that you must follow your heart and do what is best for you, your family, and your furry loved ones.

Thank you for reading Chapter Six because a healthy pet is a happy pet. My top suggestions for pet beds and blankets can be found in the resource section of this book.

Conclusion

I believe firmly that to help make this world a better place, we must respect Mother Earth. Know that our magnificent God created this beautiful planet out of His love for us. We need to play our part in doing all that we can to take good care of her. Partaking in more organically sourced ingredients, using less toxic products, and growing as much of our food as we can are essential ways we can live in harmony with nature.

If we live and love in sync with the Earth, the Earth will live in sync with us. Respecting and caring for animals is one important aspect of making the world a better, happier place. All animals want is a warm, loving home, with good food, toys, positive interaction with humans and other animals, and lots of love.

Losing a pet can be one of the most painful situations you will ever go through, and no other animal can ever take their place—but please, extend that love and love again. Open your heart and bless another furry baby. Love is eternal and that love can be passed on instead of held inside. We are all one, connected through love.

The righteous man cares for the needs of their animals, but the kindest acts of the wicked are cruel.

Proverbs 12:10 (NIV)

Resource Section

Foods and Treats

BobsRedMill.com
Castorpolluxpet.com
Instinctpetfood.com
K9granolafactory.com
Newmansown.com
Nummytumtum.com
Onedegreeorganics.com
Thehonestkitchen.com

Raw Honey

Reallyraw.com
Ysorganic.com

Nut Butters

Artisanaorganics.com
Vivapura.com

Coconut, Olive, Hempseed and Red Palm Oils and Hemp Seeds

Gardenoflife.com
Nutiva.com

Supplements

Bixbi.com
Gardenoflife.com

Hawaiipharm.com
Herbsmithinc.com
Maryruthorganics.com
Organictraditions.com
Petsbynature.com
Petwellbeing.com
Solidgoldpet.com
Vimergy.com
Zestypaws.com

Pet Detox Products

Animalessentials.com
Hawaiipharm.com
Petwellbeing.com

Toys

Koashouse.com
Olivegreendog.com
Westpaw.com

Beds and Blankets

Olivegreendog.com
Mercolomarket.com

Bath Products and Bug Repellent

Cedarcide.com
Davismfg.com
Earthanimal.com
Earthbath.com

Pet Brushes and Tick Removers

Ecotradecompany.com
Furbliss.com
Packagefreeshop.com

Nail Clippers

Onlynaturalpet.com

Ear Cleaners for Dogs and Cats

Vetorganics.com

About the Author

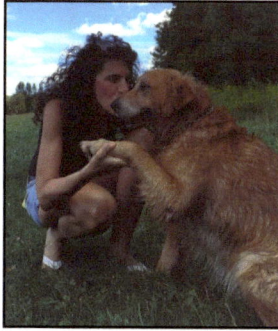

Tonijean Kulpinski, BCHP AADP, is a Certified Biblical Health Coach, and a Board-Certified Holistic Drugless Practitioner. She is also a member of The American Association of Drugless Practitioners.

It is her life's passion and purpose to transform the health of both humans and animals through the truth revealed in God's pharmacy. Tonijean lives with her loving husband Vladimir, her beautiful daughter Michaela, and her precious English cream golden retriever, Milky Way—and fur-ever in her heart, her beloved golden retriever, Peanut.

Notes

Notes

Notes

www.ingramcontent.com/pod-product-compliance
Lightning Source LLC
Chambersburg PA
CBHW040513290326
41930CB00035B/7